ENDOMETRIOSIS DIET PLAN

A Beginner's 3-Week Step-by-Step Guide for Women, With Curated Recipes and a Sample Meal Plan

Mary Golanna

mindplusfood

CONTENTS

DISCLAIMER

By reading this disclaimer, you are accepting the terms of the disclaimer in full. If you disagree with this disclaimer, please do not read the guide.

All of the content within this guide is provided for informational and educational purposes only, and should not be accepted as independent medical or other professional advice. The author is not a doctor, physician, nurse, mental health provider, or registered nutritionist/dietician. Therefore, using and reading this guide does not establish any form of a physician-patient relationship.

Always consult with a physician or another qualified health provider with any issues or questions you might have regarding any sort of medical condition. Do not ever disregard any qualified professional medical advice or delay seeking that advice because of anything you have read in this guide. The information in this guide is not intended to be any sort of medical advice and should not be used in lieu of any medical advice by a licensed and qualified medical professional.

The information in this guide has been compiled from a variety of known sources. However, the author cannot attest to or guarantee the accuracy of each source and thus should not be held liable for any errors or omissions.

You acknowledge that the publisher of this guide will not be held

INTRODUCTION

D id you know that the older a woman gets, the more health risks she has? Certain conditions can affect a woman mentally, emotionally, and physically. One of these factors is the food eaten.

Some conditions call for specific diet planning, for example, one of which is this condition called endometriosis. Endometriosis affects about 11% of women each year. Studies carried out show that 50% to 60% of women experience pelvic pain along with the condition.

As women grow older, the strength of their immune system weakens and can only be maintained through healthy living. This is no to say that men aren't at risk too. However, it is very rare to see a man with endometriosis. It is also known to be incurable, but that doesn't mean you can't do anything about it.

This clinical condition is common. To further handle this condition, keep reading to know more about endometriosis and how to develop a proper diet for this condition.

In this guide you will learn:

• What endometriosis is

• Causes and stage

• The best diet plan for endometriosis

- What foods to avoid if you have the condition

- How to plan and maintain a healthy 3-week diet

Although it can become problematic if left untreated, having endometriosis is not a kiss of death. A proper diet can help maintain a healthy level and reduce pelvic pain.

This guide aims to give relevant information to women with endometriosis and guide them on preparing the best endometriosis diet plan recipes that would help boost their immune systems.

ALL ABOUT ENDOMETRIOSIS

E ndometriosis is an incurable health condition that affects women especially those in their 30s and 40s. This disease refers to the growth of endometrial tissues—the parts that form a lining around the inside of the uterus—outside of the uterus.

It is characterized by severe pelvic pain and can cause infertility. This is because the uterus, ovaries, and lower abdomen are affected.

The endometrium tissue is an important factor that contributes to a woman's monthly bleeding. So the problem arises when, instead of growing inside the uterus, it grows outside it. It could grow in the ovaries, the intestines, or the fallopian tubes.

When the endometrium tissue breaks, it causes swells and pains because there is nowhere for the blood to pass through. On rare occasions, the tissue grows in the bladder, the vulva, or the cervix.

Contrary to what people think, endometriosis is not cancerous. However, if not well treated, the swelling expands to block your fallopian tubes which will cause inflammation and intestinal problems.

It is still uncertain as to what causes this disease. But most researchers have stated some possible causes like the following:

This is the first likely cause of endometriosis—although all of the causes are just based on theories and haven't been proven yet. It happens when the menstrual blood flows through the fallopian tubes and into the pelvic region, instead of passing away from the body.

For a long time, both retrograde menstruation and endometriosis have been closely linked together, but researchers are still skeptical about this cause. This is because, on very rare occasions, men with estrogen hormones are likely to get it.

2. Genetic Disposition

Researchers have been able to treat endometriosis in patients down to their family ancestors. If members of your family have a history of the condition then you are at a higher risk of getting it. It is a very likely cause, especially in families where the genes are very strong.

It is presumed by doctors and researchers that a dysfunction in the immune system is likely to cause endometriosis. A dysfunctional immune system may fail to identify and eliminate any irregular endometrial tissue that is growing outside the uterus.

Endometriosis can start with a sharp pain in the pelvic region. The pain is similar to menstrual cramps because it affects the lower abdomen and lower back too.

Pain in the pelvic region usually comes during ovulation, when passing urine, or during the period around your menstrual flow. Aside from the pain, other symptoms include:

- Heavy or irregular bleeding

- Swollen abdomen - mostly during menstruation because that is when the endometrial tissues break and the blood is stuck in the abdomen instead of passing through.

- Diarrhea, or in most cases, constipation

- Stress and fatigue, accompanied by pain

- Infertility

In the case of infertility, it is more of an effect than a symptom. Also, it is still undergoing research because most women with endometriosis have been able to get pregnant and give birth. It is just that it may be a bit difficult compared to women without the condition.

Although endometriosis and infertility are closely related, 20 to 25% of patients are asymptomatic. Also, infertile women are over four times more likely to have endometriosis, and women with endometriosis are very likely to be fertile.

According to Women's health, you are likely to get endometriosis if you:

- have menstrual periods that last for more than a week

- come from a family with an endometriosis history

- never had any biological children

- have abnormal menstrual flow

While the causes of endometriosis are still unclear and can most likely happen to anyone, experts are able to determine the four stages of this disease. The disease is divided into stages, making it easier for doctors to diagnose its severity.

Some of the classifications known were by the American Society for Reproductive Medicine (ASRM), the ENZIAN, and the EFI.

The most popular classification is that of the revised ASRM, and it is also the most accepted. It gives a well-detailed description of the severity and location of the pain. It is classified according to the number of endometriotic lesions it has and the severity of the scar tissue.

Stage 1 (minimal) — the number of implants or scar tissues is few and superficial. It has a total of 1–5 points.

Stage 2 (mild) — the implants increase in number and become deeper. It is between 6–15 points.

Stage 3 (moderate) — the implants become many and filmy adhesions begin to form. There is a presence of small cysts on the ovaries. It scores between 16–40 points.

Stage 4 (severe) — this is the final stage of the disease. It marks any points that are greater than 40 and it is very severe. It has many deep implants with larger cysts on the ovaries. The adhesions become very dense and increase in number.

Note that the stages do not relate to the level of pain felt. For example, A woman with stage 1 endometriosis doesn't mean that she feels less pain than the other one with stage 3.

Doctors do not immediately diagnose endometriosis in women; it takes about 3 to 11 years to be fully diagnosed with the disease. This is because the symptoms are similar to other health conditions.

To officially diagnose a patient as having the disease, doctors have to perform a procedure called laparoscopy. It involves making a small incision in the abdomen and using a light and camera, which is attached to a thin tube, to view the area of pain and check for any endometrial tissue. The thin tube is called a laparoscope.

This is what helps them to identify the stage of the disease by using the ASRM staging system. Laparoscopy can also be used to remove any visible endometriosis implant or cyst on the ovary—if there is any. However, that doesn't mean it will cure the disease.

Another reason for the delay in diagnosing endometriosis is normalizing painful and abnormal menstruation. Sometimes, the symptoms will be dismissed as chronic menstrual cramps, more commonly known as dysmenorrhea, and treated as such.

Most women diagnosed with endometriosis first noticed symptoms during their teenage years. Late diagnosis could lead to more complications. Thus, it is important to visit your doctor regularly for a check-up if the pain persists.

BEST DIET FOR ENDOMETRIOSIS

Endometriosis is incurable and unpreventable. However, you can either manage it or lower your chances of it worsening. It is possible to manage the pain and also manage it from spreading and going to a higher stage. You can do so through the following:

● Medical treatment — taking painkillers, hormone therapy, hysterectomy (removal of the uterus and ovaries), and laparoscopy.

● Natural process — maintaining a specific diet to help boost the immune system and drastically reduce the pain.

While you can engage in simple activities—such as taking warm baths, doing exercise regularly, and resting—to reduce the pain, the more recommended approach is the nutritional approach. This includes developing and maintaining a healthy endometriosis diet plan that is both safe and natural.

A healthy diet contains healthy vitamins and minerals that boost the immune system and helps manage pain. Before taking up any diet, it is advisable to consult your doctor to know if you have any allergies, so you can prevent any underlying health risks that may occur.

You should avoid foods that boost your estrogen hormone. Your diet plays a very vital role in endometriosis because it can either trigger the symptoms or manage them to a minimal level.

There are several ways to get a healthy diet plan, but the two effective special diets are a Gluten-Free Diet (GFD) and a FODMAP diet.

Just like the name says, you have to go gluten-free. This means that your diet must not contain any food with gluten. This is because gluten contributes to endometrial pain—so typically, GFD reduces the painful symptoms. It helps keep the pain at a minimum or manageable level.

FODMAP aims to help the gastrointestinal system. It involves cutting out carbohydrates from your entire diet. The carbohydrates include processed foods, dairy products, added sugars, and of course, gluten.

An endometriosis diet plan would help you keep track of what you have been eating and let you know if you are on the right track. However, it is very advisable to consult your doctor or dietician before going ahead with your diet plan.

Both diets are very good, but for the sake of this guide, we would be focusing on the gluten-free diet plan because it is more better and effective than the FODMAP diet.

As earlier stated, a diet is said to be gluten-free if it contains absolutely no trace of gluten. Gluten refers to the proteins found in wheat, rye, and barley. It is the general name for these proteins, so it is right to say that pasta, bread, cereal, and any flour-produced product, including cake, contain gluten.

When compared to a FODMAP diet, GFD is more effective because it contains more nutrients. The FODMAP diet requires that you cut off dairy products. On the other hand, the GFD allows non-gluten dairy products, which contain even more nutrients.

Research has shown that a lot of people are gluten intolerant because of celiac disease. Because of this, bakeries are now producing gluten-free options. Gluten intolerance can cause the following:

• Digestion problems, like bloating, abdominal pain, inflammation, constipation

• Fatigue, anxiety, numbness, and confusion

• Weight loss, headache, and anemia

• Skin-related problems, like eczema and rash

These effects contribute heavily to the pain and discomfort of endometriosis. There is an increase in gluten-free diets, so it won't be difficult to create a diet plan.

Take note that on its own, gluten is not unhealthy. It is just that most people are increasingly becoming intolerant.

For a healthy GFD, your diet plan should include:

• Meat and fish

• Plain diary

• Gluten-free starch and flour

• Fruits and vegetables because they are naturally gluten-free

• Seeds and nuts like walnuts, almonds, and cashew

• Beverages

• Grains like rice, corn, millet, and gluten-free oats.

The gluten-free diet plan would help reduce chronic pelvic pain and inflammation by relieving you of any digestive problems like constipation and bloating. A perfect endometriosis diet plan must contain:

● Iron-rich foods to help reduce the effect of the heavy bleeding

● Fiber — from a diet of nuts, vegetables, gluten-free oats, fruits, and so on

● Vitamin B foods — like green vegetables, broccoli, cauliflower, cabbage, kale, and horseradish

● Omega fatty acids from oily fish like salmon, seeds, and tree nuts

These foods are very rich in nutrients and should form the key ingredients of your diet plan. If you want to increase your chances of fertility, even though you have endometriosis, drink enough water. It is best to keep yourself hydrated. Dehydration can cause more pain and fatigue than you can imagine.

Each of the foods that must be contained in an endometriosis diet plan has a major effect on the condition.

1. Iron-rich foods

Foods like red meat, beans, seafood, spinach, and any food that is high in iron are recommended. These foods are rich in potassium, magnesium, and folic acid. They help strengthen the bones and the immune system.

However, red meat should be taken in very limited portions. For example, 1-2 servings per week. Too much red meat can cause hormone imbalance, which could lead to inflammation and increase pelvic pain.

These foods contain lots of vitamins and are rich in both flavonoids and carotenoids. They also have anti-inflammatory properties. Fiber foods contribute to a healthy digestive tract and help keep blood sugar at a normal level.

This includes fruits, vegetables, nuts and seeds, and whole grains. The number of servings you should take, so consult your doctor/dietician to get more insights. When choosing fruits, make sure to choose only organic fruits. Inorganic fruits contain high levels of pesticides which would be detrimental to your health.

Foods like green vegetables are very rich in vitamins A, E, and C. These foods ensure that you have your daily dose of vitamins which the body may lack due to the condition. Vegetables are also rich in anti-inflammatory and antioxidant properties.

Oily fish like Alaskan salmon, sardines, herring, and including nuts and seeds, are very rich in Omega 3. Omega 3 is anti-inflammatory, which helps to dramatically reduce any inflammation that may occur. Also, vegetable oils are rich in Omega 3 and contain high levels of monounsaturated fat that causes good cholesterol.

5. Lean meat and eggs

They are low in saturated fat. Saturated fat contributes unhealthy cholesterol to the body.

6. Low-fat dairy products

Foods like low-fat cheese, skim milk, and fat-free yogurt contain vitamin D and help reduce the number of hormones (especially estrogen) in your diet.

Consumption of processed foods or soft drinks is dangerous because they contain high inflammatory properties.

GETTING STARTED ON THE ENDOMETRIOSIS DIET PLAN–WEEK 1

Having looked at what an ideal endometriosis diet plan should consist of in the previous chapter, you probably have an idea of recipes to include in your diet plan but do not know how to start.

However, as stated at the beginning of this guide, you will be shown a step-by-step guide on how to start your 3-week diet plan with some sample recipes you can easily prepare in a short amount of time and how to prepare them.

Remember, these are just samples to guide you in preparing your recipe. You can create any recipe you want but make sure they don't contain any ingredient that is dangerous and can worsen the condition. You can also follow these samples too because they have been approved by a top dietician.

We know how difficult it is to practice GFD. Here is a step-by-step guide to help you get used to GFD. Do not fret. Be hopeful and stay motivated in the fact that it only takes 21 days, exactly 3 weeks, to develop a habit.

The goal of this step-by-step guide is to help you get acquainted with the diet. You don't have to dive in just like that, there is a high tendency that you would give up easily.

It takes a process to completely get acquainted with the diet plan. In no further ado, here is the step-by-step process:

As the first step to a gluten-free diet plan, get rid of ALL gluten products in your house. Right from your fridge to your kitchen cabinets, and medicine cabinet, dispose of or donate all food ingredients containing gluten. Such as:

• Wheat-based foods

• Barley

• Rye

• Triticale (cross between wheat and rye)

• Malt

• Brewer's yeast

Also, do not forget to clean out your medicine cabinet and remove gluten-containing cosmetics, toothpaste, vitamins, supplements, and pharmaceutical drugs. Since wheat starch is usually used in tablets and capsules as a binding agent.

You can ask your doctor or dermatologists if there are other gluten-free alternatives to your favorite cosmetics, toothpaste, or medicine brands.

If you are extremely sensitive to the smallest amount of gluten, we encourage you to replace regularly used kitchen tools like your frying pan and cooking utensils.

Here is a checklist to avoid cross-contamination with your gluten-free food:

☑ Replace the toaster and only use it for gluten-free bread

☑ Replace cooking pans with stainless steel

☑ Replace ovenware or place a foil or parchment paper

☑ Replace dishwashing materials

☑ Purchase a new non-porous chopping board

☑ Have a separate storage area for gluten-free food

During this period, you can start introducing gluten-free food into your diet at least once a day. Practice cooking them yourself at home. Do this by starting to include some of the gluten-free products, mentioned in the previous chapter, to your grocery shopping list.

WEEK 1 SAMPLE
RECIPES

Arugula and Mushroom Salad

Ingredients:

- 5 oz. arugula washed
- 1 lb. fresh mushrooms
- 1/4 tsp. shoyu
- 1/2 red onion
- 1 tbsp. olive oil
- 1 tbsp. mirin

For tofu cheese:

- 1/8 cup umeboshi vinegar
- 1/2 firm tofu

Instructions:

1. In a bowl, add the rinsed tofu. Crumble and pour in vinegar.

2. In a separate bowl add shoyu, red onions, salt, olive oil, and mirin. 3. Mix to combine.

4. Add in the arugula and toss to combine with the dressing.

5. Serve and enjoy.

Avocado, Cucumber, and Tomato Salad

Ingredients:

- 1/4 cup extra-virgin olive oil
- 1 pc. lemon, juiced
- 1/4 tsp. cumin, ground
- salt, to taste
- freshly ground black pepper, to taste
- 3 medium avocados, cubed
- 1-pint cherry tomatoes, halved
- 1 small cucumber, sliced into half-moons
- 1/3 cup corn
- 2 tbsp. cilantro, chopped

Instructions:

1. Combine avocados, cilantro, corn, cucumber, jalapeño, and tomatoes in a large bowl.

2. In a separate small container, whisk together lemon juice, cumin, and oil to make the salad dressing.

3. Season the dressing with salt and pepper.

4. Toss the salad gently while adding the dressing.

5. Serve immediately.

JUST FRESH PRODUCE AND MEAT–WEEK 2

A t this point, it is not safe yet to explore processed gluten-free foods. Since you have yet to learn how to identify what is gluten-free from what claims to be gluten-free.

To keep it simple, stick first with meat and fresh produce. They are usually found on the sides of the supermarket. This should be at the top of your grocery shopping list.

Plan your meals ahead of time and your grocery list should consist of ingredients you promise to stick to while doing your grocery shopping. This will also help in avoiding unnecessary calories from alternatives and from developing nutritional deficiencies.

If you have existing comorbid diseases and nutritional deficiencies, it is suggested you seek consultation with a dietician first before finalizing your grocery list. In fact, your entire grocery list has to be reviewed by your dietician to ensure that you are on the right track.

Once in the grocery, skip the sections for junk and processed food. Not only will you get to save money, but you will also be able to save up so much time. Make sure to only go for organic produce and less red meat. Inorganic produce can contain toxic substances that are harmful to your health, while too much red meat can increase inflammation and worsen the condition.

Take note, having a diet plan prepares you for the transition journey, from gluten to non-gluten. With this, you also have an idea of what food you are eating next.

WEEK 2 SAMPLE RECIPES

Chicken Salad

Ingredients:

- 1 small can of premium chunk chicken breast packed in water
- 1 stalk celery, large, finely chopped
- 1/4 cup reduced-fat mayonnaise
- 4 romaine leaves or red leaf lettuce, washed and trimmed
- 8 pcs. cherry tomatoes or 1 ripe tomato, quartered
- 1 cucumber, small and sliced thinly

Instructions:

1. Drain canned chicken and transfer to a bowl.
2. Put in celery and mayonnaise.
3. Mix lightly. Don't crush the chicken.
4. In a separate shallow bowl, place the lettuce neatly.
5. Add the chicken salad in the middle
6. Add tomatoes and cucumber slices to the plate.
7. Refrigerate before serving, cover with plastic wrap.

Egg Salad with Avocados

Ingredients:

- 3 medium-sized avocados
- 6 eggs, large and hard-boiled
- 1/3 red onion, medium size
- 3 celery ribs
- 4 tbsp. mayonnaise
- 2 tbsp. freshly squeezed lime juice
- 2 tsp. brown mustard
- 1/2 tsp. cumin powder
- 1 tsp. hot sauce
- salt
- pepper

Instructions:

1. Chop the eggs, celery, and onion.

2. Set aside the avocados, then combine the rest of the ingredients.

3. Slice the avocado in half to take out the pit.

4. Stuff the avocado by spooning the egg salad on its cave.

5. Serve and enjoy.

PRACTICE DISTINGUISHING GLUTEN-FREE PRODUCTS–WEEK 3

In the previous chapter, you should already be getting acquainted with just the fresh produce and meat available at the grocery store. Now, it's time to explore the processed food section in the supermarket. Find time to look for gluten-free labels by the FDA.

There are ingredients and products in the market that claim to be gluten-free but still contain some amounts of hidden gluten. Beware of products that include the following as part of their ingredients:

- Hydrolyzed malt extract
- Triticum aestivum
- Secale cereale (rye)
- Hydrolysate
- Dextrin

- Triticum vulgare (wheat)

- Vitamin E yeast extract

- Brown rice syrup

- Hydrolyzed soy protein

- Fermented grain extracts

The above ingredients are code names for gluten. Make sure to always look at the ingredients before adding any item to the shopping cart.

According to the Food and Drug Administration, under the Food Allergen Labeling and Consumer Protection Act of 2004 (FALCPA), foods labeled "gluten-free" should only contain 20 parts per million (ppm) gluten per kilogram of food or less.

Look closely and double-check if there is any hint of gluten in the list of ingredients. The common ones would be milk, eggs, and wheat.

Since you still need to watch your nutrition, stay away from complicated labels. Usually, the longer the label, the more processed it is.

The following are some examples of gluten-free food and ingredients broken down carefully in a table for you to easily remember:

Basic food	Grains and starch-containing food:	Beverages:
1. Fruits 2. Vegetables 3. Meat and poultry 4. Fish and seafood 5. Dairy 6. Beans, legumes, and nuts	1. Rice 2. Cassava 3. Corn 4. Potato 5. Soy 6. Tapioca 7. Sorghum 8. Quinoa 9. Millet 10. Buckwheat groats 11. Amaranth 12. Arrowroot 13. Teff 14. Flax 15. Chia 16. Yucca 17. Gluten-free oats	Most beverages are gluten-free, but it's safer to always check the labels.

More of this list is in "Gluten Free Food List | IBS Diet." For more guidelines on the recommended daily intake, you may refer to Nutrient Recommendations: Dietary Reference Intakes (DRI).

Get a diet plan journal, where you can keep track of all the foods you have prepared for the entire week. Include also any changes you may have noticed so far. This will help you identify which recipes work and which don't.

WEEK 3 SAMPLE RECIPES

Vegetable Broth

Ingredients:

- 1 tbsp. oil
- 2 leeks, sliced
- 2 carrots, sliced
- 2 ribs celery
- 1/4 tsp. salt
- 8 cups water

To make the soup:

- 1 tbsp. oil
- 2 cups potatoes, diced
- 1 cup mushrooms, diced
- 1-1/2 cups cauliflower, diced
- 1 cup onion, diced
- 1 cup celery, diced
- 1 cup carrot, diced
- 1-1/2 cups red beans, cooked
- 2 sprigs rosemary
- 4 sprigs thyme
- 2 cups spinach

Instructions:

1. To a pot on medium heat, add oil and leeks.
2. Cook for about three minutes or until they start to soften up.

3. Add carrots and top a few celery stalks with leaves.

4. Cover with water.

5. Add salt. Bring to a simmer and cook until carrots are very tender but not mushy.

6. Turn off the heat and let it cool down a little.

7. When the broth has cooled down, strain out the veggies.

8. Remove carrots and set them aside.

9. Squeeze most of the liquid out of the leeks and celery.

To cook the soup:

1. Add carrots to some of the broth and blend.

2. With a pot on medium heat, add oil, onions, raw carrots, and celery. Cook until onions are translucent, approximately 3 to 5 minutes.

3. Add broth, potatoes, and herbs.

4. Bring to a simmer and cook for 10 minutes.

5. Add cauliflower and red beans.

6. Simmer for another 5 minutes.

7. Add the package of frozen green beans and cook until the potatoes and cauliflower are tender, approximately for another 5 minutes.

8. At the end of cooking, add spinach.

9. Serve warm.

Salmon Salad

Ingredients:

- 2 large filets of wild salmon, either poached or grilled and then chilled
- 1 cup cherry tomatoes, halved
- 2 red onions, sliced
- 1 tbsp. balsamic vinegar
- 1 tbsp. capers
- 1 tbsp. fresh dill, finely chopped
- 1 tbsp. extra-virgin olive oil
- 1/4 tsp. pepper, freshly ground
- salt

Instructions:

1. Remove skin and bones from the cooled salmon.
2. Break salmon into chunks, and place them into a bowl.
3. Add tomatoes, red onion, and capers. Toss ingredients.
4. Combine balsamic vinegar, olive oil, and dill in a separate bowl.
5. Pour the mixture over the salmon chunks. Toss again.
6. Sprinkle it with salt and pepper to taste.
7. Chill salad for at least half an hour before serving.

BONUS STEP: JOIN SUPPORT GROUPS, EAT OUT AND SOCIALIZE

Now you have identified gluten-free products and have gotten used to them as being part of your daily life, it is to socialize. By socializing, it's joining endometriosis support groups where you can ask questions about the condition and the diet, and meet other people that are just like you. Joining a support group helps you sustain this new lifestyle and gives you the strength you will need as you get to know that you are not alone in your journey.

Having an endometriosis diet plan doesn't mean you are forbidden to eat out. As long as you can now identify gluten-free products, you can eat out—only ordering the option with gluten-free ingredients. Always ask if the meal you are about to order is gluten-free. Or if the staff is not knowledgeable enough, ask for the ingredients. It is always better to ask and be sure than assume and regret later on.

ADDITIONAL
SAMPLE RECIPES

Spinach and Chickpeas

Ingredients:

- 3 tbsp. extra virgin olive oil
- 1 onion, thinly sliced
- 4 cloves garlic, minced
- 1 tbsp. grated ginger
- 1/2 container grape tomatoes
- 1 lemon, zested and freshly juiced
- 1 tsp. crushed red pepper flakes
- 1 large can of chickpeas
- 6 cups spinach
- sea salt

Instructions:

1. Add extra virgin olive oil to a large skillet, add onion, and cook until the onion starts to brown.

2. Add all the ingredients except for the chickpeas. Cook for 3 to 4 minutes.

3. Add cooked chickpeas and stir. Add oil if necessary.

4. Serve and enjoy.

Zucchini and Celery Greens Soup

Ingredients:

- 1/2 cup cooked green lentils
- 1 onion, finely diced
- 1 parsnip, peeled and finely diced
- 2 garlic cloves, crushed
- 1 green bell pepper, cut into small cubes
- 1 zucchini, sliced
- 4 asparagus spears
- 1 fennel bulb, diced finely
- 2 celery stalks, diced finely
- 1 small bunch of celery greens or other greens available: beet greens, kale, or spinach
- 2 cups low sodium vegetable broth
- 1 lime, juice only
- 1 tsp. chia seeds to garnish
- freshly ground black pepper

Instructions:

1. Stir-fry onion and garlic, about 2 minutes.

2. Throw in the parsnip, bell pepper, fennel, celery stalks, and zucchini, along with the vegetable broth.

3. Wait until it boils. Then, lower the heat and let it simmer for 7 minutes.

4. Put in the asparagus, lime juice, lentils, and celery greens. Turn off the heat.

5. Serve warm, garnished with chia seeds.

Seafood Stew

Ingredients:

- 2 tsp. extra-virgin olive oil
- 1 cut bulb fennel
- 2 stalks celery, chopped
- 2 cups white wine
- 1 tbsp. chopped thyme
- 1 cup chopped shallots
- 6 ounces shrimp
- 6 ounces of sea scallops
- 1/4 tsp. salt
- 1 cup chopped parsley
- 6 oz. Arctic char
- 2-1/2 cups of water

Instructions:

1. Heat a frying pan on the lowest setting. Add a small amount of oil.

2. Cook the celery, shallots, and fennel for approximately 6 minutes.

3. Pour the wine, water, and thyme into the frying pan.

4. Wait for 10 minutes and allow it to cook.

5. Once much of the water has evaporated, add in the remaining ingredients, and wait for 2 minutes before removing it from the stove.

6. Serve and enjoy immediately.

Pine Nut Quinoa Bowl

Ingredients:

• 1 cup dry white quinoa

Marinara sauce:

• 1-1/4 tbsp. agave nectar

• 1/4 cup extra-virgin olive oil, preferably cold-pressed

• 2 cups sun-dried tomatoes, water-soaked for a couple of hours

• 2 tbsp. lemon juice

• 1 cup soaking water used for tomatoes

• 1/2 yellow onion, chopped

• 2 large heirloom or Roma tomatoes, diced

• 1 handful fresh basil leaves, reserve some for garnish

• 3-4 garlic cloves, crushed

• 1 tsp. sea salt

• 2 tsp. dried oregano

• 1/4 cup pine nuts, reserve some for garnish

• a pinch of hot pepper flakes

Instructions:

To cook the quinoa:

1. Wash quinoa.

2. Boil quinoa with 2 cups of filtered water in a medium saucepan.

3. Reduce heat to low and let it simmer.

4. Cover and cook for about 15 to 20 minutes. The quinoa must be

tender and fluffy and has absorbed all the water.

To make the marinara sauce:

1. Put all the marinara sauce ingredients in a high-speed blender.

2. Blend everything for about 30-45 seconds, or until smooth. Mix with a tamper in between to help with the blending.

3. Optional: To thin out the sauce, use the water you used to soak the tomatoes and pour it into the blender.

4. Optional: Set the sauce to simmer at a low temperature in a medium saucepan for 25 to 30 minutes.

5. Upon serving, pour a spoonful of the marinara sauce over the cooked quinoa.

6. Top with pine nuts and fresh basil leaves.

7. Serve immediately.

HOW TO LIVE WITH ENDOMETRIOSIS

Having endometriosis doesn't mean it is the end of the world for you. Endometriosis may be a chronic illness but with proper management and the right diet, you can live with it like every other normal person.

Not only do you have to keep your diet in check, but you also have to keep your mental health in check. It is no news that the most troubling symptoms of endometriosis are pain and infertility.

Studies have shown that infertility is the most dreadful symptom of endometriosis and the most difficult aspect. Dealing with fertility issues can be a devastating period for both you and your close family members. For this reason, it is very advisable to go through counseling sessions to help ease your stress mentally and emotionally.

Although infertility is like a 50:50 chance, experts say that the best way to get used to fertility issues—if they ever come—is with time. There is a popular saying that goes "Time heals the deepest wounds," and infertility is not an exception.

Learning to live with endometriosis is a process. At first, it may seem like a struggle to cope with your daily life. The first reaction, immediately after diagnosis, is usually fear, anxiety, and disbelief. Over time, you would begin to be more concerned about gathering more information about the condition and how to go about the right treatment process.

Maintaining a consistent healthy endometriosis diet plan keeps the symptoms of endometriosis at their barest minimum. This is because endometriosis is an inflammatory disease and you need to take in more anti-inflammatory properties to reduce the pain.

Ways to cope with endometriosis include:

• Being faithful to your diet plan

• Using a heating pad to reduce pelvic pain

• Staying hydrated. Water should be part of your diet plan

• Keeping a daily journal for tracking all your daily activities

• Maintaining a healthy lifestyle, no drinking or smoking

• Meditating and exercising often to reduce stress

• Scheduling counseling appointments with your doctor, dietician, and therapist

• Surrounding yourself with family, friends, and support groups

CONCLUSION

E ndometriosis is an incurable illness that affects about 11% of women each year. This means that it is a common illness and that you are not alone. For some women, the pain is usually unbearable due to the inflammation and swelling of the pelvic region.

However, what you eat or don't eat plays a very big role in your endometriosis journey. If in doubt about any diet plan or recipe, it is best to consult your doctor or dietician.

Thank you again for getting this guide. If you found this guide helpful, please take the time to share your thoughts and post a review. It would be greatly appreciated!

Thank you and good luck on your journey!

REFERENCES AND HELPFUL LINKS

8 easy steps to kick gluten to the curb—Permanently. (n.d.). Verywell Fit. Retrieved December 16, 2022, from https://www.verywellfit.com/how-to-go-gluten-free-563172.

Ballard K, Lowton K, Wright J. What's the delay? A qualitative study of women's experiences of reaching a diagnosis of endometriosis. Fertil Steril 2006; 86(5):1296–1301.

Carpan, Ann Carolyn (1996) Learning to live with endometriosis: a grounded theory study. Masters thesis, Memorial University of Newfoundland.

endometriosis.org. (n.d.). Causes – Endometriosis.org. Retrieved December 16, 2022, from https://endometriosis.org/endometriosis/causes/.

Food and Drug Administration, HHS. (2013). Food labeling: Gluten-free labeling of foods. Final rule. Federal Register, 78(150), 47154–47179.

Giudice, L. C. (2010). Clinical practice. Endometriosis. The New England Journal of Medicine, 362(25), 2389–2398. https://doi.org/10.1056/NEJMcp1000274.

Gluten free food list. (n.d.). IBS Diets. Retrieved December 16, 2022, from https://www.ibsdiets.org/ibs/gluten-free-food-list/.

Gluten-free foods. (n.d.). Celiac Disease Foundation. Retrieved December 16, 2022, from https://celiac.org/gluten-free-living/gluten-free-foods/.

Hudelist G, Fritzer N, Thomas A, et al. Diagnostic delay for endometriosis in Austria and Germany: causes and possible consequences. Hum Reprod 2012; 27(12):3412–3416.

Husby GK, Haugen RS, Moen MH. Diagnostic delay in women with pain and endometriosis. Acta Obstet Gynecol Scand. 2003 Jul;82(7):649-53. doi: 10.1034/j.1600-0412.2003.00168.x. PMID: 12790847.

Journal of the American dietetic association 108 (4), 661-672, 2008.

Marziali M, Venza M, Lazzaro S, Lazzaro A, Micossi C, Stolfi VM. Gluten-free diet: a new strategy for management of painful endometriosis-related symptoms? Minerva Chir. 2012 Dec;67(6):499-504. PMID: 23334113.

Office of dietary supplements—Nutrient recommendations and databases. (n.d.). Retrieved December 16, 2022, from https://ods.od.nih.gov/HealthInformation/nutrientrecommendations.aspx.

Revised American Society for Reproductive Medicine. Classification of endometriosis: 1996. American Society for Reproductive Medicine.

Savaris AL, do Amaral VF. Nutrient intake, anthropometric data, and correlations with the systemic antioxidant capacity of women with pelvic endometriosis. Eur J Obstet Gynecol Reprod Biol. 2011; 158:314-8.

The beginners guide to going gluten free | best in gluten free. (n.d.). Schär. Retrieved December 16, 2022, from https://www.schaer.com/en-us/a/how-go-gluten-free-beginners.

Verkauf, B. S. (1987). Incidence, symptoms, and signs of endometriosis in fertile and infertile women. The Journal of the Florida Medical Association, 74(9), 671–675.

Weinstein, K. (1987). Living With Endometriosis: How to Cope With the Physical and Emotional Challenges. Massachusetts: Addison-Wesley Publishing Company, Inc.